Cancer Diet Cookbook for Women Over 50

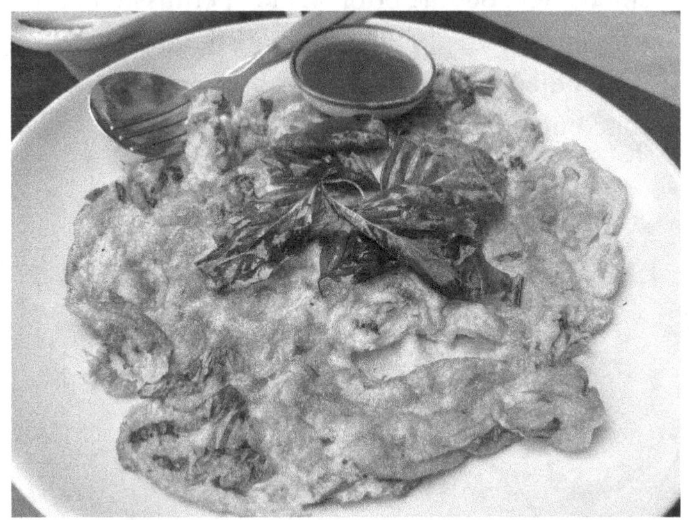

An Ultimate Guide to Quick and Easy Nourishing Anticancer Recipes for Cancer Prevention, Treatment and Recovery

Grace C. Whitford

TABLE OF CONTENTS

Introduction

Embark on a transformative journey towards a healthier, more conscious lifestyle specifically tailored for women navigating their 50s. In this guide, we plunge into the intricacies of a cancer-conscious diet, offering profound insights, statistical revelations, and practical counsel to empower you as you navigate the path to holistic well-being.

Illuminating the Significance of a Cancer-Conscious Diet for Women Over 50

As women traverse the landscape of their 50s, they encounter profound shifts in hormonal dynamics, ushering in an era where health concerns, notably cancer, become more prevalent. The significance of embracing a cancer-conscious diet during this life stage cannot be overstated. Our dietary choices wield remarkable influence over cellular functions, hormone equilibrium, and the body's ability to ward off potential cancer threats.

This section takes a deep dive into the nuanced reasons underpinning the criticality of a cancer-conscious diet for women over 50. By unraveling the intricate connection between nutrition and cancer, we aim to elucidate how specific dietary nuances can play a pivotal role in both preventing and managing the complexities of cancer.

Unveiling Statistics on Cancer Prevalence in Women Over 50

Equipping ourselves with an understanding of the prevalence of cancer among women in their 50s is instrumental in fostering awareness and instigating proactive health measures. Recent statistics underscore a heightened vulnerability to breast, ovarian, and colorectal cancers within this demographic. Delving into these statistics serves as a catalyst for women to embrace early detection methods, adopt transformative lifestyle changes, and, significantly, recognize the indispensable role that dietary choices play in mitigating the risk of these cancers.

In this section, we aim to unfold the layers of these statistics, shedding light on the profound implications they carry. Through this, we empower women with knowledge, encouraging informed decisions about their health, and cultivating a sense of agency over their well-being.

Unraveling the Intricacies of Nutrition in Cancer Prevention and Management

In the quest for cancer prevention and management, nutrition emerges as a formidable ally. This segment conducts a thorough exploration of the specific nutrients, antioxidants, and bioactive compounds inherent in certain foods, all scientifically proven to curtail cancer risk and bolster overall health.

Our journey takes us into the inner workings of how nutrition operates at a cellular level, influencing critical factors such as inflammation, oxidative stress, and hormonal equilibrium. By comprehending the intricate interplay between individual dietary choices and the body's cellular landscape, women over 50 can make informed decisions, fortifying their defenses against the intricate dance of cancer pathways.

This introductory chapter lays a sturdy foundation for our comprehensive exploration of cancer-conscious nutrition for women over 50. As we navigate through subsequent chapters, anticipate gaining not just knowledge but practical insights, expert guidance, and a personalized meal plan crafted to embolden your journey toward optimal health and sustained well-being

Chapter 1

Understanding Cancer and Nutrition

Welcome to the immersive exploration of "Cancer Diet Cookbook for Women Over 50." In this comprehensive chapter, we will embark on a profound journey to unravel the intricate relationship between cancer and nutrition. Our goal is to equip you with a deep understanding of how dietary choices can influence cancer risk and progression. By delving into the profound impact of key nutrients and antioxidants on cancer prevention, and providing practical guidance on foods to include and avoid for a cancer-conscious diet, we aim to empower you with knowledge that extends beyond the pages of this cookbook.

As we navigate through the realms of science and culinary artistry, our collective aim is to not only nourish your body but also to empower you with the knowledge required to make informed choices that positively impact your health. Together, let us embark on a transformative journey towards embracing a vibrant, well-balanced life.

Explanation of How Diet Can Influence Cancer Risk and Progression

Cancer, an intricate and multifaceted disease, is influenced by a multitude of factors, and among these, diet plays a pivotal role in both the susceptibility to cancer and the trajectory of the disease. This section aims to provide an in-depth exploration of the intricate relationship between dietary choices and cancer, shedding light on the mechanisms through which the foods we consume intricately impact cellular processes, inflammation, and the body's ability to defend against cancerous cells.

1. Orchestrating Cellular Processes Through Nutrient Influence:

At the core of our being lie trillions of cells, each perpetually engaged in the ballet of growth, division, and renewal. Nutrients derived from our diet are the conductors orchestrating these cellular processes. Specific dietary elements, ranging from essential vitamins to minerals and antioxidants, assume critical roles in safeguarding the integrity of our genetic material and steering the meticulous progression of cell cycles.

2. Unraveling the Dynamics of Inflammation in Cancer Development:

Chronic inflammation emerges as a significant player in the genesis and advancement of various cancer types. Certain dietary choices, particularly those high in saturated fats, refined sugars, and processed meats, contribute to the inflammation milieu within the body. This persistent inflammatory environment becomes a fertile ground for the growth and sustenance of cancer cells. Conversely, embracing an anti-inflammatory diet abundant in fruits, vegetables, and omega-3 fatty acids may potentially dampen the inflammatory response, thus reducing the risk of cancer development.

3. Antioxidants as Vigilant Cellular Custodians:
In the complex tapestry of cellular life, antioxidants stand as vigilant custodians against oxidative stress. Abundant in fruits, vegetables, and whole grains, antioxidants serve as defenders against the onslaught of free radicals—unstable molecules capable of damaging cellular structures, including DNA. By neutralizing these free radicals, antioxidants fortify the body's defense against cellular damage, forming a robust barrier against the potential onset of cancer.

4. The Dance of Dietary Choices and Hormonal Balance:
The impact of dietary patterns on hormonal equilibrium cannot be understated, especially concerning hormone-related cancers like breast and prostate cancer. A diet rich in saturated fats may contribute to hormonal imbalances, while a diet abundant in fiber sourced from fruits, vegetables, and whole grains may play a regulatory role. Actively managing and understanding these hormonal influences through dietary choices becomes a proactive strategy in mitigating cancer risk.

5. Microbiome Harmony and Its Potential Influence on Cancer:

Within the intricate ecosystem of the digestive tract resides the gut microbiome, emerging as a key player in overall health, including its potential sway over cancer susceptibility. Current research suggests that the composition of the microbiome may influence inflammation, immune responses, and even the metabolism of specific nutrients. Dietary choices, such as the inclusion of fiber-rich foods and probiotics, can positively shape the microbiome, fostering an environment conducive to overall health and potentially diminishing the risk of specific cancers.

6. Weight Management as a Crucial Factor in Cancer Prevention:

Strategically managing weight through mindful dietary choices and an active lifestyle emerges as a critical facet of cancer prevention. Obesity, a known risk factor for various cancers including breast, colorectal, and pancreatic cancer, underscores the importance of dietary patterns that encourage weight management. A balanced diet comprising nutrient-dense foods alongside regular physical activity contributes not only to weight regulation but also significantly diminishes the risk of cancers associated with obesity.

In summary, the intricate interplay between diet and cancer risk and progression unfolds across various dimensions. Armed with knowledge and making thoughtful dietary decisions, individuals can actively participate in reducing their vulnerability to cancer and promoting overall well-being. This foundational understanding sets the stage for the ensuing chapters of this cookbook, seamlessly translating this knowledge into practical, delectable recipes meticulously crafted for the well-being of women over 50 navigating the complexities of cancer.

Key Nutrients and Antioxidants Essential for Cancer Prevention

Within the intricate weave of cancer prevention, the spotlight shines brightly on key nutrients and antioxidants, serving as integral elements that fortify the body against the initiation and progression of cancer. This section aims to delve into the depths of these crucial components, unraveling the profound impact they wield in empowering individuals to make informed dietary choices that contribute to holistic well-being.

1. Vitamin C: A Defender Against Oxidative Stress
Vitamin C, renowned for its antioxidant prowess, stands as a formidable guardian against oxidative stress—a precarious imbalance capable of triggering cellular damage and fostering the environment for cancer initiation. Found abundantly in citrus fruits, strawberries, and bell peppers, the integration of vitamin C-rich foods becomes a powerful strategy to fortify the body's natural defenses, enhancing its resilience against the complexities of cancer.

2. Selenium: Tracing the Path of Antioxidant Power
Selenium, a trace mineral possessing potent antioxidant properties, takes center stage in the prevention of certain cancers. Abundant in nuts, seeds, and seafood, selenium serves as a critical player in neutralizing free radicals and regulating DNA synthesis and repair. By incorporating selenium-rich foods, individuals embark on a journey to enhance cellular defenses, creating an environment less conducive to the initiation of cancerous processes.

3. Glucosinolates in Cruciferous Vegetables: A Potent Arsenal

Cruciferous vegetables, such as broccoli, cauliflower, and Brussels sprouts, boast a potent arsenal of cancer-fighting compounds known as glucosinolates. These compounds, upon digestion, give rise to bioactive substances associated with reduced cancer risk. The inclusion of these cruciferous champions in one's diet not only provides a flavorful culinary experience but also serves as a robust nutritional strategy for cancer prevention.

4. Polyphenols in Green Tea and Turmeric: An Antioxidant Symphony

Green tea, rich in polyphenols, has earned acclaim for its potential cancer-preventive properties. The antioxidant effects of green tea catechins play a role in mitigating oxidative stress and inflammation. Similarly, turmeric, with its active compound curcumin, boasts anti-inflammatory and antioxidant properties. Integrating green tea and turmeric into the diet not only introduces delightful flavors but also offers a potent boost to the body's defense mechanisms against cancer.

5. Omega-3 Fatty Acids: Balancing the Equation

Abundant in fatty fish like salmon and flaxseeds, omega-3 fatty acids contribute to a comprehensive strategy for cancer prevention. These essential fatty acids, recognized for their anti-inflammatory properties, regulate cellular function and may impede the growth of cancer cells. Embracing sources of omega-3 fatty acids in the diet presents a harmonious balance aligning with the body's innate defenses.

6. Antioxidant-Rich Fruits and Vegetables: A Spectrum of Protection

The vivid palette of fruits and vegetables mirrors a rich spectrum of antioxidants, actively combating free radicals. From the carotenoids in carrots and sweet potatoes to the anthocyanins in berries, each pigment represents a unique set of antioxidants. Embracing a diverse array of colorful fruits and vegetables ensures a comprehensive intake of antioxidants, fortifying the body's defense against oxidative stress and championing overall health.

7. Vitamin D: A Multifaceted Sunshine Nutrient

Vitamin D, often hailed as the "sunshine vitamin," assumes a multifaceted role in cancer prevention. While sunlight serves as a natural source, dietary contributions from fatty fish, fortified dairy, and supplements maintain optimal vitamin D levels. Research suggests that vitamin D influences cell growth regulation and immune function, providing protective effects against specific cancers.

8. Fiber: Guardian of Digestive Health

Dietary fiber, abundant in whole grains, fruits, and vegetables, emerges as a stalwart guardian of digestive health with implications for cancer prevention. A high-fiber diet promotes regular bowel movements, reducing the duration of harmful substance interaction with the intestinal lining. Additionally, fiber fosters a healthy gut microbiome, supporting digestive well-being and potentially diminishing the risk of colorectal cancer.

The incorporation of these key nutrients and antioxidants into the daily diet signifies a proactive stance toward cancer prevention. As individuals embark on this gastronomic expedition, the vibrant hues and diverse flavors on their plates symbolize not only a delightful meal but also a commitment to nourishing the body with essential elements that fortify its resilience against the intricate landscape of cancer. Subsequent chapters of this cookbook will seamlessly integrate these insights into practical and delectable recipes, tailored to empower women over 50 in their pursuit of holistic well-being.

Foods to Include and Avoid for a Cancer-Conscious Diet

Embarking on a journey toward a cancer-aware diet involves not only understanding what to include but also being mindful of what to exclude. This section offers an in-depth exploration of the foods that should be part of your dietary repertoire, as well as those that are best left off the plate, forming a robust framework for a proactive approach to cancer prevention.

Foods to Embrace:

1. Rainbow of Fruits and Vegetables:

- **Inclusions:** Incorporate a spectrum of colors with berries, citrus fruits, leafy greens, and cruciferous vegetables.

- **Rationale:** These vibrant options bring a plethora of vitamins, minerals, and antioxidants, fortifying cellular health and combating oxidative stress, potentially reducing the risk of diverse cancers.

2. Wholesome Grains:

- **Inclusions:** Opt for quinoa, brown rice, oats, and whole wheat.

- **Rationale:** Rich in fiber, these whole grains provide sustained energy, support digestive health, and may contribute to lowering the risk of colorectal cancer.

3. Lean Proteins:

- **Inclusions:** Choose fish, poultry, tofu, and legumes.

- **Rationale:** Lean protein sources offer essential amino acids without the saturated fats present in red and processed meats, potentially lowering the risk of specific cancers.

4. Healthy Fats:

- **Inclusions:** Enjoy avocado, nuts, seeds, and olive oil.

- **Rationale:** Monounsaturated and polyunsaturated fats provide a source of energy without the detrimental effects associated with saturated fats, supporting heart health.

5. Probiotic-Rich Foods:

- **Inclusions:** Integrate yogurt, kefir, sauerkraut, and kimchi.

- **Rationale:** Probiotics foster a healthy gut microbiome, enhancing digestive health and potentially reducing the risk of colorectal cancer.

6. Green Tea Elixir:

- **Inclusions:** Sip on green tea.

- **Rationale:** Abundant in polyphenols, green tea exhibits antioxidant properties that may help mitigate oxidative stress and reduce the risk of certain cancers.

7. Cruciferous Powerhouses:

- **Inclusions:** Embrace broccoli, cauliflower, Brussels sprouts, and kale.

- **Rationale:** Packed with glucosinolates, these vegetables are associated with a reduced risk of certain cancers, including breast and prostate cancer.

8. Stay Hydrated:

- **Inclusions:** Prioritize water and herbal teas.

- **Rationale:** Adequate hydration supports overall health, aids digestion, and promotes the elimination of toxins from the body.

Foods to Approach with Caution:

1. Processed Meats:
   - **Exclusions:** Limit intake of bacon, sausages, and deli meats.
   - **Rationale:** Processed meats often contain preservatives and additives that may contribute to an increased risk of colorectal cancer.

2. Sugary Beverages:
   - **Exclusions:** Minimize consumption of soda, energy drinks, and sugary fruit juices.
   - **Rationale:** High sugar intake is linked to obesity and an increased risk of various cancers, including breast and colorectal cancer.

3. Red and Processed Meats:
   - **Exclusions:** Reduce consumption of beef, pork, and processed meats.
   - **Rationale:** High intake of red and processed meats is associated with an elevated risk of colorectal cancer.

4. Saturated Fats:
   - **Exclusions:** Limit consumption of fried foods, fatty cuts of meat, and full-fat dairy.

- **Rationale:** Diets high in saturated fats may contribute to inflammation and an increased risk of certain cancers.

5. Excessive Alcohol:

- **Exclusions:** Moderation in alcohol consumption.
- **Rationale:** Excessive alcohol intake is linked to an elevated risk of certain cancers, including breast, liver, and colorectal cancer.

6. Refined Carbohydrates:

- **Exclusions:** Minimize intake of white bread, pastries, and sugary cereals.
- **Rationale:** High consumption of refined carbohydrates may lead to weight gain and an increased risk of obesity-related cancers.

7. High-Salt Foods:

- **Exclusions:** Limit processed foods, canned soups, and salty snacks.
- **Rationale:** High-salt diets have been linked to an increased risk of stomach cancer.

8. Trans Fats:

   - **Exclusions:** Avoid trans fats found in margarine and commercially baked goods.

   - **Rationale:** Trans fats, common in processed and fried foods, may contribute to inflammation and an increased risk of certain cancers.

Crafting a cancer-aware diet involves thoughtful considerations and a balanced approach to food choices. By emphasizing nutrient-dense foods and minimizing the intake of potentially harmful substances, individuals can actively contribute to their overall well-being and reduce the risk of cancer. This comprehensive foundation will guide the development of delectable and health-supporting recipes in the subsequent chapters, tailored specifically for women over 50 navigating the challenges of cancer.

Chapter 2

Tailoring the Diet to Women Over 50

As we transition into the heart of our culinary exploration, we find ourselves at a pivotal juncture—Chapter 2, where our focus shifts towards the distinctive needs of women over 50. This chapter, "Tailoring the Diet to Women Over 50," transcends a mere section; it serves as a bespoke guide crafted to navigate the nuanced landscape of nutrition for women entering a remarkable phase of life.

Within these pages, we embark on an in-depth exploration of the specific nutritional requirements, hormonal transitions, and health considerations that accompany this age group. Recognizing that a one-size-fits-all approach falls short, we embark on a journey of customization, acknowledging that the choices made in the kitchen play a pivotal role in supporting vitality and well-being for women navigating the golden years.

From dissecting the unique nutritional needs of this demographic to unraveling the impact of hormonal changes on dietary preferences, this chapter unfolds as a compass guiding us toward nourishment that resonates with the wisdom and experience that define women over 50. It's an invitation to embrace the intersection of taste and wellness, where each recipe becomes a celebration of life's rich tapestry.

As we tailor our culinary endeavors to meet the distinctive needs of women over 50, let's approach this chapter with anticipation, ready to discover the flavors and nutrients that harmonize with the vibrancy and grace characterizing this incredible stage of life. Subsequent sections will unfurl a menu meticulously curated with precision, presenting delectable dishes that align seamlessly with the unique dietary considerations of women over 50. Together, let's savor the essence of personalized nutrition, celebrating health, wisdom, and the joy of a well-nourished life.

Nutritional Needs Specific to Women in their 50s

Embarking on the journey through life entails a dynamic dance with hormonal fluctuations, influencing the multifaceted aspects of health and well-being. For women, especially those in their 50s, the onset of menopause introduces a spectrum of hormonal changes that wield profound effects on both physical and physiological dimensions. A nuanced understanding of these hormonal shifts and their intricate influence on diet emerges as a cornerstone for cultivating a nourishing and supportive approach to overall wellness.

1. **Estrogen Decline and its Metabolic Implications:**
   - **Context:** The menopausal phase witnesses a decline in estrogen levels, instigating notable changes in metabolism.
   - **Impact on Diet:** Adapting caloric intake and focusing on nutrient-dense foods assumes significance as metabolism undergoes a potential slowdown. The incorporation of lean proteins, whole grains, and an array of fruits and vegetables emerges as a strategic move to bolster metabolic health.

2. Estrogen's Role in Bone Health:

- **Context:** Estrogen plays a pivotal role in preserving bone density, and its reduction during menopause heightens the risk of osteoporosis.

- **Impact on Diet:** Prioritizing dietary sources rich in calcium, such as dairy and fortified plant-based alternatives, along with ensuring adequate vitamin D intake, becomes imperative to fortify and maintain optimal bone health.

3. Hormonal Effects on Insulin Sensitivity and Blood Sugar Regulation:

- **Context:** Hormonal fluctuations can influence insulin sensitivity, thereby impacting blood sugar regulation.

- **Impact on Diet:** The adoption of a diet characterized by complex carbohydrates, fiber-rich foods, and mindful sugar consumption emerges as a strategy to stabilize blood sugar levels. Consistent, balanced meals contribute to sustained energy throughout the day.

4. Weight Distribution and Hormonal Influence:

- **Context:** Hormonal changes may dictate alterations in fat distribution, often resulting in weight gain, particularly around the abdominal region.

- **Impact on Diet:** The inclusion of omega-3 fatty acid-rich foods, such as fatty fish and flaxseeds, alongside regular physical activity, stands as a proactive measure for managing weight and promoting cardiovascular health.

5. Emotional Well-being in the Face of Hormonal Flux:

- **Context:** Hormonal fluctuations can contribute to mood swings and emotional shifts.

- **Impact on Diet:** Prioritizing foods abundant in serotonin precursors, like proteins containing tryptophan and complex carbohydrates, emerges as a dietary approach that positively influences mood. Additionally, maintaining a well-balanced diet fosters overall emotional well-being.

6. Hormonal Impact on Muscle Maintenance:

- **Context:** Hormonal shifts may influence muscle mass, introducing the risk of sarcopenia.

- **Impact on Diet:** Ensuring an adequate intake of protein sourced from lean meats, poultry, fish, dairy, and plant-based alternatives becomes instrumental in supporting muscle maintenance and overall strength.

7. Gut Health and Hormonal Harmony:

   - **Context:** Hormonal changes can exert an influence on gut health and digestive patterns.

   - **Impact on Diet:** The prioritization of fiber-rich foods, encompassing whole grains, fruits, and vegetables, stands as a dietary pillar fostering digestive health and mitigating common concerns like constipation.

8. Hormones' Role in Skin Health:

   - **Context:** The decline of estrogen can impact skin elasticity and hydration.

   - **Impact on Diet:** The integration of antioxidant-rich foods, spanning a spectrum of colorful fruits and vegetables, delivers essential nutrients that support skin health and counteract oxidative stress.

Comprehending the nuanced interplay between hormonal changes and dietary choices equips women in their 50s with the knowledge to traverse this phase with resilience and informed decision-making. Crafting a diet that aligns with these hormonal shifts contributes not only to physical health but also plays a pivotal role in supporting emotional and mental well-being. In subsequent chapters, these insights will seamlessly integrate into practical and delectable recipes, tailored to resonate with the unique needs of women over 50 experiencing transformative hormonal changes.

Tailoring Nutrition to the Unique Needs of Women in Their 50s

Entering the fifth decade of life is a transformative period for women, characterized by distinct physiological changes that necessitate a nuanced approach to nutrition. Catering to the nutritional needs specific to women in their 50s becomes essential in supporting overall health, managing hormonal shifts, and mitigating the risk of age-related health issues. This section comprehensively explores the critical facets of dietary requirements for women navigating this pivotal stage of life.

1. Caloric Intake and Metabolism:
   - **Context:** The natural decline in metabolic rate and lean muscle mass, coupled with hormonal changes, can contribute to weight gain in women in their 50s.
   - **Strategic Approach:** Prioritize nutrient-dense foods, emphasizing lean proteins, whole grains, fruits, and vegetables. Mindful portion control becomes crucial to support metabolic health.

2. Calcium and Bone Health:
   - **Context:** Postmenopausal women face an increased risk of osteoporosis due to declining estrogen levels affecting bone density.
   - **Strategic Approach:** Ensure an ample intake of calcium-rich foods such as dairy, leafy greens, and fortified plant-based alternatives. Vitamin D supplementation and sunlight exposure are pivotal for calcium absorption.

3. Iron and Anemia Risk:
   - **Context:** With the cessation of menstrual cycles, iron loss decreases but the risk of iron overload may rise. Iron absorption from plant-based sources tends to diminish with age.
   - **Strategic Approach:** Incorporate lean meats, fortified cereals, and vitamin C-rich foods to

enhance iron absorption. Regular monitoring of iron levels is advisable.

4. Protein Intake and Muscle Maintenance:

- **Context:** Sarcopenia, the age-related loss of muscle mass, becomes a concern, necessitating adequate protein intake for muscle maintenance.

- **Strategic Approach:** Prioritize protein-rich foods including lean meats, poultry, fish, dairy, legumes, and plant-based sources to fortify muscle health and overall strength.

5. Heart Health and Omega-3 Fatty Acids:

- **Context:** Postmenopausal women face an increased risk of heart disease, emphasizing the importance of omega-3 fatty acids in reducing cardiovascular risk.

- **Strategic Approach:** Incorporate sources of omega-3 fatty acids such as fatty fish (salmon, mackerel), flaxseeds, chia seeds, and walnuts to promote heart health.

6. Fiber for Digestive Health:

- **Context:** Aging can contribute to digestive issues, and hormonal changes may impact bowel regularity.

- Strategic Approach: Prioritize fiber-rich foods like whole grains, fruits, vegetables, and legumes to support digestive health and prevent constipation.

7. Antioxidants and Skin Health:

- Context: Aging can affect skin elasticity and hydration, emphasizing the role of antioxidants in protecting the skin from oxidative stress.

- Strategic Approach: Integrate a diverse array of fruits and vegetables rich in antioxidants, such as berries, citrus fruits, and leafy greens, to support skin health and combat oxidative damage.

8. Hydration and Kidney Function:

- Context: Aging kidneys may experience decreased function, impacting fluid balance.

- Strategic Approach: Maintain optimal hydration through water and hydrating foods like fruits and vegetables. Limiting caffeine and alcohol intake is advisable to support kidney health.

Recognizing and addressing these specific nutritional needs for women in their 50s is a proactive step toward maintaining health, vitality, and resilience in the face of age-related changes. Customizing the diet to meet these requirements ensures a foundation of well-being that encompasses physical, mental, and emotional aspects—a holistic approach to embracing and celebrating this significant stage of life.

Hormonal Changes and their Impact on Diet

Embarking on the journey through life entails a dynamic dance with hormonal fluctuations, influencing the multifaceted aspects of health and well-being. For women, especially those in their 50s, the onset of menopause introduces a spectrum of hormonal changes that wield profound effects on both physical and physiological dimensions. A nuanced understanding of these hormonal shifts and their intricate influence on diet emerges as a cornerstone for cultivating a nourishing and supportive approach to overall wellness.

1. **Estrogen Decline and its Metabolic Implications:**

- **Context:** The menopausal phase witnesses a decline in estrogen levels, instigating notable changes in metabolism.

- **Impact on Diet:** Adapting caloric intake and focusing on nutrient-dense foods assumes significance as metabolism undergoes a potential slowdown. The incorporation of lean proteins, whole grains, and an array of fruits and vegetables emerges as a strategic move to bolster metabolic health.

2. **Estrogen's Role in Bone Health:**

- **Context:** Estrogen plays a pivotal role in preserving bone density, and its reduction during menopause heightens the risk of osteoporosis.

- **Impact on Diet:** Prioritizing dietary sources rich in calcium, such as dairy and fortified plant-based alternatives, along with ensuring adequate vitamin D intake, becomes imperative to fortify and maintain optimal bone health.

3. **Hormonal Effects on Insulin Sensitivity and Blood Sugar Regulation:**

- **Context:** Hormonal fluctuations can influence insulin sensitivity, thereby impacting blood sugar regulation.

- **Impact on Diet:** The adoption of a diet characterized by complex carbohydrates, fiber-rich foods, and mindful sugar consumption emerges as a strategy to stabilize blood sugar levels. Consistent, balanced meals contribute to sustained energy throughout the day.

4. Weight Distribution and Hormonal Influence:

- **Context:** Hormonal changes may dictate alterations in fat distribution, often resulting in weight gain, particularly around the abdominal region.

- **Impact on Diet:** The inclusion of omega-3 fatty acid-rich foods, such as fatty fish and flaxseeds, alongside regular physical activity, stands as a proactive measure for managing weight and promoting cardiovascular health.

5. Emotional Well-being in the Face of Hormonal Flux:

- **Context:** Hormonal fluctuations can contribute to mood swings and emotional shifts.

- **Impact on Diet:** Prioritizing foods abundant in serotonin precursors, like proteins containing tryptophan and complex carbohydrates, emerges as a dietary approach that positively influences mood. Additionally, maintaining a well-balanced diet fosters overall emotional well-being.

6. Hormonal Impact on Muscle Maintenance:

- **Context:** Hormonal shifts may influence muscle mass, introducing the risk of sarcopenia.

- **Impact on Diet:** Ensuring an adequate intake of protein sourced from lean meats, poultry, fish, dairy, and plant-based alternatives becomes instrumental in supporting muscle maintenance and overall strength.

7. Gut Health and Hormonal Harmony:

- **Context:** Hormonal changes can exert an influence on gut health and digestive patterns.

- **Impact on Diet:** The prioritization of fiber-rich foods, encompassing whole grains, fruits, and vegetables, stands as a dietary pillar fostering digestive health and mitigating common concerns like constipation.

8. Hormones' Role in Skin Health:

- **Context:** The decline of estrogen can impact skin elasticity and hydration.

- **Impact on Diet:** The integration of antioxidant-rich foods, spanning a spectrum of colorful fruits and vegetables, delivers essential nutrients that support skin health and counteract oxidative stress.

Comprehending the nuanced interplay between hormonal changes and dietary choices equips women in their 50s with the knowledge to traverse this phase with resilience and informed decision-making. Crafting a diet that aligns with these hormonal shifts contributes not only to physical health but also plays a pivotal role in supporting emotional and mental well-being. In subsequent chapters, these insights will seamlessly integrate into practical and delectable recipes, tailored to resonate with the unique needs of women over 50 experiencing transformative hormonal changes.

Addressing Common Health Concerns in this Age Group Through Diet

As women gracefully step into their 50s, a tapestry of health considerations unfolds, demanding a diet tailored to address these unique challenges. Developing a nutritional strategy that proactively tackles these common health concerns emerges not only as a wise choice but as a fundamental aspect of nurturing comprehensive well-being. This section meticulously explores key health considerations, unraveling how dietary choices can serve as a cornerstone in mitigating risks and promoting optimal health for women in this age group.

1. Cardiovascular Health:

- **Concern:** Postmenopausal women face an elevated risk of cardiovascular issues.

- **Dietary Strategy:** Prioritize heart-healthy foods rich in omega-3 fatty acids from fatty fish, whole grains abundant in fiber, and an array of fruits and vegetables. Restricting saturated fats and sodium intake forms a foundational pillar in sustaining cardiovascular health.

2. Bone Health and Osteoporosis:

- **Concern:** Diminished estrogen levels increase susceptibility to osteoporosis.

- **Dietary Strategy:** Elevate calcium intake through dairy, fortified plant-based alternatives, and vitamin D sources. Augmenting nutritional support with weight-bearing exercises further bolsters bone health.

3. Weight Management:

- **Concern:** Hormonal fluctuations and a sluggish metabolism contribute to weight gain.

- **Dietary Strategy:** Embrace a balanced diet teeming with lean proteins, whole grains, and a profusion of fruits and vegetables. The amalgamation of portion control and consistent physical activity forms a dynamic duo in the realm of weight management.

4. Hormonal Balance and Menopausal Symptoms:

- **Concern:** Menopausal symptoms, encompassing hot flashes and mood swings, disrupt daily life.

- **Dietary Strategy:** Integrate phytoestrogen-rich foods like soy products and flaxseeds to potentially alleviate menopausal discomfort. Sustaining stable blood sugar levels through well-balanced meals contributes to mood stability.

5. Digestive Health:

- **Concern:** Aging introduces shifts in digestive patterns.

- Dietary Strategy: Prioritize a wealth of fiber from whole grains, fruits, and vegetables to champion digestive health. The inclusion of probiotic-rich foods like yogurt and kefir fosters a thriving gut microbiome.

6. Cognitive Health and Memory Concerns:

- Concern: Cognitive well-being takes center stage, with apprehensions about memory and cognitive decline.

- Dietary Strategy: Infuse the diet with antioxidants found in berries and leafy greens to champion brain health. Incorporating omega-3 fatty acids from sources like fatty fish and walnuts potentially contributes to cognitive function.

7. Type 2 Diabetes Risk:

- Concern: Aging and metabolic shifts elevate the risk of type 2 diabetes.

- Dietary Strategy: Opt for complex carbohydrates, curtail added sugars, and prioritize low glycemic index foods. Vigilant monitoring of blood sugar levels and maintaining a healthy weight form integral components of diabetes risk management.

8. Hydration and Kidney Function:
- **Concern:** Aging kidneys may experience diminished function.
- **Dietary Strategy:** Ensure optimal hydration through water and hydrating foods. A judicious limit on caffeine and alcohol intake emerges as a supportive measure for kidney health.

By strategically navigating these common health concerns through a purposeful diet, women in their 50s can fortify their bodies, optimize health outcomes, and savor a holistic sense of well-being. The ensuing chapters of this cookbook seamlessly weave these principles into tantalizing recipes, presenting a practical and enjoyable pathway to embrace a health-conscious lifestyle finely tuned for the distinctive needs of women in this vibrant and transformative age group.

Chapter 3

Creating a Cancer Diet Plan

In this pivotal chapter of "Cancer Diet Cookbook for Women Over 50," our focus turns to the practical intricacies of translating nutritional principles into a daily culinary experience. Here, we embark on a comprehensive journey, providing profound insights into weekly meal planning, the significance of portion control, and the artistry of integrating a diverse array of cancer-fighting foods. We aim to cultivate a harmonious and sustainable approach to nourishment, one that not only supports overall well-being but also caters to the unique nutritional needs of women over 50 facing the challenges of cancer.

Weekly Meal Planning Guide

1. Mastering the Essentials of Meal Planning:
Effective meal planning forms the bedrock of a well-rounded cancer-conscious diet. Let's navigate through a systematic guide to aid you in this process:

- **Tailoring to Dietary Needs:** Initiate the planning process by understanding individual dietary needs, considering factors such as age, weight, medical conditions, and personal preferences.

- **Diversity in Nutrients:** Strive for a diverse range of nutrients, encompassing proteins, carbohydrates, healthy fats, vitamins, and minerals. This diversity supports overall health and caters to specific nutritional demands during cancer treatment.

- **Macronutrient Harmony:** Maintain a delicate balance of proteins, carbohydrates, and fats in each meal, fostering sustained energy levels and supporting various bodily functions.

- **Strategic Meal Timing:** Distribute meals and snacks throughout the day, considering energy levels, appetite, and any treatment-related side effects. Align meal timing with medical treatments or medication schedules.

2. Practical Tips for Weekly Meal Planning:

- **Efficient Batch Cooking:** Optimize your time and effort by preparing larger quantities of select meals, allowing for freezing and subsequent use. This not only saves time but also ensures a repository of nutritious options.

- **Embrace Seasonal and Local Ingredients:** Prioritize seasonal and locally sourced produce for optimal freshness and nutritional content. This approach not only promotes health but also aligns with sustainability ideals.

- **Flexibility in Plans:** Acknowledge that plans may require adjustments based on energy levels, appetite, and potential treatment-related side effects. Embrace adaptability while maintaining a commitment to balanced nutrition.

- **Consider Family Preferences:** Account for the preferences of family members, creating an inclusive meal environment. Adjust flavors and textures to suit diverse tastes.

Portion Control and Balanced Nutrition

1. Unlocking the Power of Portion Control:

- **Personalized Portions:** Tailor portions to individual energy needs and health objectives, acknowledging that everyone's requirements are unique.

- **Guarding Against Overeating:** Smaller, more frequent meals can prevent overeating and help manage digestive symptoms commonly associated with cancer treatments.

- **Listening to Body Signals:** Foster mindful eating by paying attention to hunger and fullness cues, promoting a healthy and intuitive relationship with food.

2. Balancing Nutrition for Wholesome Well-being:

- **Prioritize Protein-Rich Foods:** Lean proteins such as poultry, fish, legumes, and tofu should take precedence to support muscle maintenance and repair, especially critical during cancer treatment.

- **Whole Grains for Sustained Energy:** Opt for whole grains like brown rice, quinoa, and whole wheat, providing a gradual release of energy and vital nutrients like fiber.

- **Embrace Healthy Fats:** Integrate sources of healthy fats such as avocados, nuts, and olive oil, crucial for overall health and aiding in the absorption of specific nutrients.

- **A Rainbow of Fruits and Vegetables:** Aim for a spectrum of colorful fruits and vegetables to harness a wide array of vitamins, minerals, and antioxidants. This diversity contributes to immune support and overall vitality.

- **Prioritize Hydration:** Ensure adequate hydration, particularly essential during cancer treatment. Water, herbal teas, and hydrating foods like soups and fruits collectively contribute to overall fluid intake.

Incorporating a Variety of Cancer-Fighting Foods

1. Decoding the Realm of Cancer-Fighting Foods:

- **Phytochemical-Rich Selections:** Opt for foods rich in phytochemicals, natural compounds found in plants with potential cancer-fighting properties. Examples include cruciferous vegetables (broccoli, cauliflower), berries, and green tea.

- **Indulge in Antioxidant Powerhouses:** Integrate antioxidant-rich foods to combat oxidative stress. Berries, dark leafy greens, nuts, and seeds are exceptional choices.

- **Harness the Benefits of Omega-3 Fatty Acids:** Include fatty fish (salmon, mackerel), flaxseeds, chia seeds, and walnuts for their anti-inflammatory properties, potentially beneficial during cancer treatment.

- **Celebrate the Colors of Fruits and Vegetables:** Consume a diverse assortment of colorful fruits and vegetables to ensure a broad spectrum of nutrients. The vibrant hues often signify the presence of valuable compounds.

2. Practical Strategies for Integration:

- **Revitalize with Smoothies and Juices:** Craft nutrient-rich smoothies or juices using a blend of fruits, vegetables, and other cancer-fighting ingredients. These concoctions serve as a convenient and delicious means of boosting nutritional intake.

- **Elevate Flavor with Herbs and Spices:** Enhance both flavor and nutritional value by incorporating herbs and spices into your meals. Turmeric, garlic, ginger, and cinnamon, for instance, offer anti-inflammatory and antioxidant benefits.

- **Embrace Plant-Based Proteins:** Infuse your diet with plant-based protein sources like legumes, tofu, and tempeh. These not only contribute to protein intake but also offer additional phytonutrients.

- **Incorporate Fermented Delights:** Integrate fermented foods such as yogurt, kefir, and sauerkraut, which contain probiotics supporting gut health—crucial during and after cancer treatment.

- **Diversify Cooking Techniques:** Experiment with various cooking methods, including roasting, steaming, and raw preparations, to retain the maximum nutritional value of foods.

In the subsequent chapters, these insights seamlessly merge into delectable recipes, ensuring that each bite becomes a deliberate step toward vitality and well-being. As we continue this culinary exploration, may your kitchen become a canvas for crafting not just meals, but a nourishing lifestyle attuned to the unique needs of women over 50 on the path to wellness.

Chapter 4

Quick and Delicious Recipes

Embark on a culinary odyssey that seamlessly merges health, flavor, and simplicity in the pages of "Cancer Diet Cookbook for Women Over 50." In this chapter, our focus transitions to crafting swift and delectable recipes meticulously curated to align with the distinctive nutritional needs of women over 50. From invigorating breakfast options to lunches bursting with nutrients and dinners that satisfy both palate and soul, each recipe is a testament to the belief that every bite can be a celebration of well-being.

Breakfast Options Promoting Health and Energy

1. Overnight Oats with Berries and Almonds:

Ingredients:
- Rolled oats
- Almond milk
- Fresh berries (blueberries, strawberries, raspberries)
- Sliced almonds
- Honey or maple syrup (optional)

Preparation:
- Combine rolled oats and almond milk in a jar.
- Add a medley of fresh berries and sliced almonds.
- Refrigerate overnight.
- Drizzle with honey or maple syrup before serving.

Health Benefits:

- Oats provide sustained energy and a hearty dose of fiber.

- Berries contribute antioxidants, while almonds add healthy fats and protein.

2. Spinach and Feta Omelette:

Ingredients:

- Eggs
- Fresh spinach
- Feta cheese
- Cherry tomatoes (optional)
- Olive oil

Preparation:

- Whisk eggs and pour into a heated, oiled pan.

- Add fresh spinach, crumbled feta cheese, and cherry tomatoes.

- Fold the omelet and cook until the eggs are set.

Health Benefits:

- Eggs offer protein and a range of essential nutrients.

- Spinach provides iron and various vitamins, while feta introduces calcium and rich flavor.

3. Greek Yogurt Parfait with Granola and Mixed Berries:

Ingredients:
- Greek yogurt
- Granola
- Mixed berries (raspberries, blackberries, strawberries)
- Honey (optional)

Preparation:
- Layer Greek yogurt, granola, and a colorful mix of berries in a glass.
- Repeat the layers.
- Drizzle with honey for added sweetness.

Health Benefits:
- Greek yogurt is a protein powerhouse with the bonus of probiotics.

- Berries contribute antioxidants and fiber, while granola introduces a delightful crunch.

4. Avocado and Smoked Salmon Bagel:

Ingredients:
- Whole grain bagel
- Smoked salmon
- Avocado slices
- Cream cheese
- Fresh dill (optional)

Preparation:
- Toast the whole grain bagel to preference.
- Spread cream cheese on the bagel halves.
- Layer smoked salmon and avocado slices.
- Garnish with fresh dill if desired.

Health Benefits:
- Whole grain bagels offer complex carbohydrates and fiber.

- Smoked salmon is rich in omega-3 fatty acids, while avocados contribute healthy fats and creaminess.

Nutrient-Rich Lunch Ideas

1. Quinoa Salad with Chickpeas and Avocado:

Ingredients:
- Quinoa
- Chickpeas (canned or cooked)
- Avocado
- Cherry tomatoes
- Fresh cilantro
- Olive oil and lemon dressing

Preparation:
- Cook quinoa and allow it to cool.
- Mix quinoa with chickpeas, diced avocado, cherry tomatoes, and chopped cilantro.

- Drizzle with olive oil and a squeeze of fresh lemon.

Health Benefits:
- Quinoa provides a complete protein source and is rich in fiber.
- Chickpeas add protein and additional fiber.
- Avocado contributes healthy fats, making this salad both nutritious and satisfying.

2. Salmon and Quinoa Bowl with Roasted Vegetables:

Ingredients:
- Salmon fillet
- Quinoa
- Assorted vegetables (bell peppers, zucchini, cherry tomatoes)
- Olive oil and balsamic glaze

Preparation:
- Roast vegetables in olive oil until tender.
- Grill or bake salmon to perfection.

- Serve over cooked quinoa and drizzle with balsamic glaze.

Health Benefits:
- Salmon offers omega-3 fatty acids for heart health.
- Quinoa is a protein-rich grain with essential nutrients.
- Assorted vegetables contribute vitamins, minerals, and fiber.

3. Mango and Shrimp Salad:

Ingredients:
- Shrimp (grilled or sautéed)
- Mixed greens
- Mango slices
- Red onion (thinly sliced)
- Cilantro
- Lime vinaigrette

Preparation:

- Arrange mixed greens on a plate.
- Top with grilled shrimp, mango slices, sliced red onion, and cilantro.
- Drizzle with a refreshing lime vinaigrette.

Health Benefits:
- Shrimp provides lean protein with a delicate flavor.
- Mango offers vitamins, antioxidants, and natural sweetness.
- The lime vinaigrette adds zesty flair without excessive calories.

4. Caprese Quinoa Bowl:

Ingredients:
- Quinoa
- Cherry tomatoes
- Fresh mozzarella
- Basil leaves
- Balsamic glaze
- Olive oil

Preparation:

- Cook quinoa and let it cool.
- Combine quinoa with halved cherry tomatoes, fresh mozzarella balls, and torn basil leaves.
- Drizzle with balsamic glaze and olive oil.

Health Benefits:

- Quinoa is a protein-rich grain with essential amino acids.
- Cherry tomatoes provide vitamins and antioxidants.
- Fresh mozzarella adds a creamy texture and calcium.

Flavorful and Satisfying Dinner Recipes

1. Lemon Garlic Baked Chicken with Roasted Vegetables:

Ingredients:
- Chicken breasts
- Lemon
- Garlic (minced)
- Assorted vegetables (carrots, broccoli, cauliflower)
- Olive oil

Preparation:
- Marinate chicken with lemon, minced garlic, and olive oil.
- Bake chicken and vegetables until golden and cooked through.
- Serve with a side of quinoa or brown rice.

Health Benefits:
- Chicken is a lean protein source.
- Lemon and garlic infuse flavor without excessive calories.

- Roasted vegetables provide vitamins, minerals, and fiber.

2. Vegetarian Stir-Fry with Tofu and Broccoli:

Ingredients:
- Tofu (extra-firm, cubed)
- Broccoli florets
- Bell peppers (sliced)
- Soy sauce
- Ginger and garlic (minced)
- Sesame oil

Preparation:
- Sauté tofu until golden.
- Add broccoli and bell peppers.
- Stir in soy sauce, minced ginger, and garlic.
- Finish with a drizzle of sesame oil.

Health Benefits:

- Tofu is a plant-based protein rich in essential amino acids.

- Broccoli provides a wealth of vitamins, antioxidants, and fiber.

- Bell peppers add color and additional nutrients to the stir-fry.

3. Eggplant and Chickpea Curry:

Ingredients:

- Eggplant (cubed)
- Chickpeas (canned or cooked)
- Coconut milk
- Curry spices (turmeric, cumin, coriander)
- Fresh cilantro

Preparation:

- Sauté cubed eggplant and chickpeas in a blend of curry spices.

- Add coconut milk and simmer until vegetables are tender.

- Garnish with fresh cilantro before serving.

Health Benefits:
- Eggplant provides fiber and antioxidants.
- Chickpeas contribute protein and additional fiber.
- Coconut milk adds creaminess with healthy fats.

4. Tomato Basil Zoodle Bowl:

Ingredients:
- Zucchini noodles (zoodles)
- Cherry tomatoes (halved)
- Fresh mozzarella balls
- Fresh basil leaves
- Balsamic glaze
- Olive oil

Preparation:
- Spiralize zucchini to create zoodles.

- Toss zoodles with halved cherry tomatoes, fresh mozzarella balls, and torn basil leaves.
- Drizzle with balsamic glaze and olive oil.

Health Benefits:

- Zucchini noodles provide a low-carb alternative with added vitamins.
- Cherry tomatoes contribute antioxidants and vitamins.
- Fresh mozzarella adds a creamy texture and a touch of calcium.

Chapter 5

Lifestyle Changes for Cancer Prevention

Welcome to a pivotal exploration into lifestyle modifications that aim to fortify and empower in "Cancer Diet Cookbook for Women Over 50." Within this chapter, we delve into a holistic approach, emphasizing the importance of regular exercise, stress management techniques, and the often overlooked yet vital role of hydration. Each lifestyle adjustment is tailored to meet the unique needs of women over 50, establishing a robust foundation for cancer prevention.

Importance of Regular Exercise

1. Unveiling the Significance of Exercise in Preventing Cancer:

Regular physical activity transcends the realm of a mere fitness routine; it emerges as a potent ally in cancer prevention. Scientific evidence consistently reveals that engaging in moderate-intensity exercise significantly diminishes the risk of various cancers. For women over 50, the benefits extend beyond prevention, encompassing enhanced immune function, improved mental health, and increased bone density.

2. Customizing Exercise to Individual Requirements:

- **Cardiovascular Exercise:** Activities like brisk walking, cycling, or swimming for at least 150 minutes weekly enhance cardiovascular health, promoting better blood flow and oxygenation.

- **Strength Training:** Integrating resistance training exercises, such as weightlifting or bodyweight exercises, maintains crucial muscle mass and bone density, vital for women in this age group.

- **Flexibility and Balance:** Yoga or tai chi, with their combination of physical postures, breath control, and meditation, offer a holistic approach to maintaining flexibility and balance.

3. Overcoming Barriers to Exercise:

- **Time Management:** Integrating short, frequent exercise sessions proves as effective as longer periods. Finding activities aligned with personal interests increases adherence.

- **Adapting to Physical Limitations:** Tailoring exercises to accommodate individual physical conditions ensures a safe and sustainable approach to fitness.

- **Social Engagement:** Participating in group activities or exercising with a friend introduces a social dimension, fostering motivation and enjoyment.

4. Incorporating Exercise into Daily Life:

- **Morning Walks:** A brisk morning walk not only kickstarts metabolism but also provides a serene setting for reflection and mindfulness.

- **Home Workouts:** Simple exercises at home, including squats, lunges, and yoga poses, require minimal equipment and offer a convenient option.

- **Dance:** Engaging in dance, whether a structured class or dancing to favorite tunes, combines exercise with enjoyment.

5. Tracking Progress and Celebrating Achievements:

- **Fitness Apps:** Utilizing technology to monitor daily activity levels, set goals, and track progress provides a tangible way to stay motivated.

- **Celebrate Milestones:** Recognizing and celebrating achievements, whether increased stamina or reaching a fitness milestone, reinforces positive behavior.

Stress Management Techniques

1. Understanding the Impact of Stress on Cancer Risk:

Chronic stress is intricately linked to an elevated risk of cancer and can exacerbate existing health conditions. For women over 50, managing stress is integral to maintaining overall well-being and mitigating its potential impact on cancer risk.

2. Incorporating Mindfulness Practices:

- **Meditation:** Mindful meditation, focusing on breath or guided imagery, promotes relaxation and reduces stress hormones.

- **Yoga:** Blending physical postures with breath control and meditation, yoga offers a holistic approach to stress management.

- **Tai Chi:** An ancient Chinese practice, tai chi combines gentle movements with deep breathing, fostering a sense of calm and balance.

3. Stress-Reducing Activities in Daily Life:

- **Nature Walks:** Spending time in nature, be it a park or a garden, has been shown to reduce stress levels and improve mood.

- **Artistic Expression:** Engaging in creative pursuits, such as painting, writing, or playing a musical instrument, provides an outlet for expression and stress relief.

- **Deep Breathing Exercises:** Simple deep breathing exercises, such as diaphragmatic breathing, can be practiced anywhere to induce a state of calm.

4. Effective Time Management:

- **Prioritizing Tasks:** Breaking tasks into manageable segments and prioritizing them reduces the feeling of being overwhelmed.

- **Setting Boundaries:** Establishing clear boundaries, both in personal and professional spheres, prevents excessive stress from external sources.

5. Building a Support System:

- **Connecting with Others:** Cultivating strong social connections and confiding in trusted friends or family members provides emotional support during challenging times.

- **Professional Guidance:** Seeking the assistance of a therapist or counselor offers strategies to cope with stressors and build resilience.

Adequate Hydration and Its Role in Cancer Prevention

1. The Crucial Connection Between Hydration and Cancer Prevention:

Adequate hydration emerges as a cornerstone of overall health, playing a pivotal role in preventing various health conditions, including cancer. For women over 50, maintaining optimal hydration levels becomes particularly significant, supporting bodily functions and mitigating potential risks.

2. Understanding Optimal Hydration:

- **Daily Water Intake:** While the general guideline suggests eight 8-ounce glasses per day, individual needs may vary based on factors such as age, activity level, and climate.

- **Balancing Fluid Sources:** Beyond water, fluid intake can include herbal teas, infused water, and hydrating foods like fruits and vegetables.

3. Hydration and Cancer Risk Reduction:

- **Detoxification:** A well-hydrated body efficiently removes toxins, potentially reducing the burden on organs and lowering cancer risk.

- **Cellular Health:** Optimal hydration supports cellular health and function, contributing to the body's ability to regulate and repair.

4. Practical Tips for Staying Hydrated:
- **Hydration Reminders:** Setting reminders or using apps to prompt regular water intake throughout the day ensures consistent hydration.
- **Infused Water:** Enhancing the flavor of water by infusing it with slices of citrus fruits, cucumber, or herbs makes hydration more enjoyable.
- **Hydrating Foods:** Incorporating water-rich foods, such as watermelon, cucumber, and oranges, into meals and snacks adds an extra layer of hydration.

5. Monitoring Hydration Status:
- **Urine Color:** Observing the color of urine can serve as a simple indicator of hydration status, with a pale yellow color generally signifying adequate hydration.
- **Thirst Response:** Responding to the body's natural thirst signals ensures timely and sufficient fluid intake.

Chapter 6

Emotional Well-being and Support

Welcome to an empathetic exploration of the emotional dimensions entwined with a cancer diagnosis in "Cancer Diet Cookbook for Women Over 50." Within this chapter, we delve into the intricacies of addressing the profound emotional impact of a cancer diagnosis, constructing a resilient support system, and embracing mindful eating practices that nurture emotional well-being. Each facet is thoughtfully interwoven into the tapestry of resilience, acknowledging the profound interplay between emotions, support, and nourishment on the healing journey.

Addressing the Emotional Impact of a Cancer Diagnosis

1. Comprehending the Emotional Landscape:
Receiving a cancer diagnosis is an earthquake that ripples through every facet of life. Women over 50, often navigating multiple roles, may find themselves wrestling with a spectrum of emotions—fear, uncertainty, and even grief. Recognizing and understanding this emotional landscape forms the initial step in fostering emotional well-being.

2. Seeking Professional Support:
- **Therapeutic Interventions:** Engaging with a therapist or counselor provides a confidential space for exploring and processing emotions.
- **Support Groups:** Participating in a cancer support group offers solace through shared experiences and the comfort of a community facing similar challenges.

3. Empowering through Education:
- **Knowledge as a Coping Mechanism:** Understanding the specifics of the diagnosis, treatment options, and potential outcomes

empowers individuals to actively engage in their care.

- **Open Communication with Healthcare Providers:** Establishing transparent communication with healthcare providers fosters a sense of partnership, reducing anxiety associated with the unknown.

4. Integrating Mind-Body Practices:

- **Mindfulness Meditation:** Cultivating mindfulness through meditation practices anchors the mind in the present moment, alleviating anxiety about the future.

- **Yoga for Emotional Balance:** Combining gentle movements, breathwork, and mindfulness in yoga becomes a powerful tool for emotional resilience.

5. Embracing Emotional Expression:

- **Journaling:** Expressing emotions through writing provides an outlet for self-reflection and emotional release.

- **Art Therapy:** Engaging in creative pursuits, such as drawing or painting, allows for non-verbal expression of emotions.

Building a Support System

1. Recognizing the Importance of Support:

Building a robust support system is not a luxury but a necessity on the journey through a cancer diagnosis. It acts as a pillar of strength, providing emotional sustenance and practical assistance.

2. Family and Friends as Anchors:

- **Open Communication:** Fostering an environment of open communication promotes understanding among family members and friends.

- **Assigning Specific Roles:** Delegating tasks and responsibilities to loved ones eases the burden on the individual undergoing treatment.

3. Community Engagement:

- **Local Support Groups:** Connecting with local support groups introduces individuals to a network of people who comprehend the unique challenges of a cancer journey.

- **Online Communities:** Virtual support communities provide a platform for seeking advice, sharing experiences, and gaining insights from individuals worldwide.

4. Professional Support Services:

- **Social Workers:** Hospital-based social workers assist in navigating practical aspects, such as insurance and transportation, alleviating logistical concerns.

- **Cancer Navigators:** Dedicated professionals guide individuals through the complex healthcare system, ensuring seamless coordination of care.

5. Self-Advocacy and Boundaries:

- **Empowering the Individual:** Encouraging self-advocacy empowers individuals to actively participate in decision-making regarding their care.

- **Setting Boundaries:** stablishing clear boundaries ensures that the support received aligns with individual needs and preferences.

Mindful Eating Practices for Emotional Well-being

1. The Interplay Between Emotions and Eating Habits:

Emotional well-being intricately intertwines with eating habits. Recognizing the connection between emotions and food choices is a crucial step toward mindful eating.

2. Cultivating Mindful Eating Habits:

- **Savoring Each Bite:** Taking time to savor and appreciate each bite fosters a deeper connection with the act of eating.

- **Listening to Hunger and Fullness Cues:** Tuning into the body's signals of hunger and fullness promotes a balanced relationship with food.

3. Nutrient-Dense Foods for Emotional Support:

- **Omega-3 Fatty Acids:** Foods rich in omega-3 fatty acids, such as fatty fish and flaxseeds, contribute to brain health and emotional well-being.

- **Complex Carbohydrates:** Whole grains and legumes provide a steady release of energy, stabilizing mood and promoting a sense of well-being.

4. Creating Rituals Around Meals:

- **Family Dinners:** Engaging in shared meals with family or friends creates a supportive and comforting environment.

- **Mindful Meal Preparation:** Taking part in the preparation of meals can be a mindful and therapeutic activity.

5. Seeking Professional Guidance:

- **Nutritional Counseling:** Consulting with a registered dietitian or nutritionist specialized in oncology provides personalized guidance.

- **Integrative Therapies:** Exploring integrative therapies, such as acupuncture or herbal supplements, under the guidance of healthcare providers, complements conventional care.

6. Balancing Indulgences and Nutritional Needs:

- **Moderation:** Allowing for occasional indulgences in favorite foods is a part of a balanced approach to eating.

- **Variety in the Diet:** Including a diverse range of nutrient-dense foods ensures the body receives essential vitamins and minerals.

Chapter 7

Tips for Shopping and Meal Preparation

Welcome to a pragmatic guide within the pages of "Cancer Diet Cookbook for Women Over 50." This chapter is a treasure trove of practical wisdom, dedicated to empowering you with insightful tips for intelligent grocery shopping, time-efficient meal preparation strategies, and the proper storage of cancer-fighting ingredients. As we embark on this culinary odyssey, these tips aim not only to simplify the process but also to elevate your ability to craft delectable, nutritionally rich meals customized for a cancer-conscious lifestyle.

Smart Grocery Shopping for Cancer-Conscious Meals

1. Curating a Nutrient-Enriched Shopping List:

- Commence with a foundation of vibrant produce: an array of vegetables and fruits, teeming with antioxidants and vitamins.

- Infuse your list with lean proteins, embracing poultry, fish, and plant-based sources like beans and legumes.

- Opt for whole grains such as quinoa and brown rice to provide sustained energy.

2. Navigating the Border of the Grocery Store:

- The store's periphery often hosts fresh produce, dairy, and proteins—abundant with whole, unprocessed foods.

- Limit forays into the central aisles, where packaged and processed foods laden with preservatives and additives abound.

3. Decoding Labels with a Discerning Eye:

- Seek products with concise ingredient lists, eschewing those laden with excessive additives or synthetic preservatives.

- Scrutinize labels for concealed sugars and opt for products with minimal sugar content.

4. Opting for Organic and Locally Sourced Selections:

- Prioritize organic produce to minimize exposure to pesticides and other chemicals.
- Explore the offerings of local farmers' markets for fresh, seasonal produce, fostering health and community ties.

5. Mindful Curation of Proteins:

- Favor lean cuts of meat and poultry to curtail saturated fat intake.
- Include fatty fish rich in omega-3 fatty acids, renowned for their anti-inflammatory prowess.

6. Embracing the Spectrum of Color and Texture:

- Select a kaleidoscope of colorful vegetables and fruits to ensure a broad spectrum of essential nutrients.
- Experiment with diverse textures and flavors to infuse meals with interest and satisfaction.

7. Infusing Culinary Creations with Cancer-Fighting Herbs and Spices:

- Integrate herbs like turmeric, ginger, and garlic into your recipes, celebrated for their anti-inflammatory and antioxidant virtues.

- Elevate flavors with fresh herbs like basil, cilantro, and parsley, enriching the taste without relying on excess salt.

Time-Saving Meal Preparation Strategies

1. Efficiency Unleashed through Batch Cooking:

- Designate a day for batch cooking staple ingredients—grains, beans, and proteins—streamlining meal assembly throughout the week.

- Leverage the power of freezing to preserve portions of prepared meals, providing convenient options on busier days.

2. Preparation and Portioning of Vegetables:

- Pre-wash, chop, and portion vegetables in advance, storing them in the refrigerator for seamless access.

- Equip your kitchen with time-saving gadgets like a vegetable chopper or mandoline for efficient preparation.

3. Harnessing the Might of Slow Cookers and Instant Pots:

- These culinary workhorses simplify the preparation of nutritious meals with minimal hands-on time.

- Utilize them for soups, stews, and one-pot dishes, allowing flavors to meld while freeing you to focus on other responsibilities.

4. Embracing One-Pan Wonders:

- Streamline cooking and minimize cleanup time with sheet pan dinners and one-pan meals.

- Combine lean proteins, vegetables, and flavorful seasonings on a single pan for a wholesome and time-efficient culinary experience.

5. Strategic Crafting of Meal Plans:

- Devise a weekly meal plan, integrating overlapping ingredients to minimize waste.

- Take note of versatile ingredients that can be repurposed across multiple recipes.

6. Snack Wisdom for Quick and Nutrient-Dense Options:

- Maintain an assortment of healthful snacks at your fingertips, including pre-cut vegetables, fresh fruit, and an array of nuts.

- Portion snacks thoughtfully to avoid overindulgence and uphold a balance of nutrition.

Proper Storage of Cancer-Fighting Ingredients

1. Optimal Refrigeration Techniques:

- Safeguard perishables like dairy, fresh produce, and cooked meals in the refrigerator to stave off spoilage.

- Organize your refrigerator to facilitate easy access to ingredients and curtail food wastage.

2. Leveraging Freezer-Friendly Containers:

- Invest in containers designed for freezing to store batch-cooked meals, soups, and sauces for extended freshness.
- Employ a labeling system indicating dates to monitor freshness and thwart freezer burn.

3. Preserving Nutritional Integrity:

- Monitor the shelf life of fresh produce, consuming it before its nutritional value diminishes.
- Consider blanching and freezing certain vegetables to lock in nutrients for prolonged use.

4. Meticulous Organization of Dry Goods:

- Store whole grains, nuts, and seeds in airtight containers to uphold freshness and deter infestation.
- Designate a specific area for dry goods, streamlining the meal preparation process.

5. Gentle Handling of Fresh Herbs:

- Envelop fresh herbs in damp paper towels and house them in airtight containers or produce bags in the refrigerator.

- Alternatively, freeze herbs in olive oil using ice cube trays for convenient portioning.

6. Vigilant Monitoring of Expiry Dates:

- Regularly inspect expiration dates on packaged items to ensure the consumption of fresh and safe ingredients.

- Implement a rotation system for pantry items, utilizing older products first to minimize waste.

Chapter 8

Understanding Supplements

Welcome to an in-depth exploration of the intricate relationship between nutrition and supplementation within the pages of "Nourish Life: A Cancer Diet Cookbook for Women Over 50." This chapter aims to provide a nuanced discussion on supplements that complement a cancer-conscious diet, stressing the importance of consulting with healthcare professionals before incorporating supplements and exploring the delicate equilibrium between whole foods and supplementation. As we traverse this terrain, our goal is to equip you with knowledge that fosters an informed and mindful approach to nourishing your body.

Discussion on Supplements that Complement a Cancer-Conscious Diet

1. Vital Nutrients and Their Natural Sources:

- **Vitamin D:** Recognized for its role in bone health, vitamin D synthesis through sunlight exposure is complemented by supplements, especially for those with limited sun access.

- **Omega-3 Fatty Acids:** While fatty fish like salmon offer a rich source, omega-3 supplements provide an additional anti-inflammatory boost.

- **Calcium:** Essential for bone health, calcium in dairy and fortified foods may require supplementation for those with specific dietary constraints.

2. Antioxidants and Immune Support:

- **Vitamin C:** Abundant in citrus fruits and peppers, vitamin C, vital for immune function, may necessitate supplements during vulnerable periods.

- **Selenium:** Found in nuts and seafood, selenium's role in immune response may prompt recommendations for supplements in cases of deficiency.

3. Herbal Supplements and Cancer Prevention:

- **Turmeric (Curcumin):** Renowned for its anti-inflammatory properties, turmeric finds a concentrated form in curcumin supplements.

- **Green Tea Extract:** Packed with antioxidants, caution is advised with supplements due to potential side effects.

4. Probiotics for Gut Health:

- **Fermented Foods:** Natural probiotics in yogurt support gut health, but supplements may be advisable for those with digestive concerns or on antibiotics.

5. Vitamin B12 for Plant-Based Diets:

- **Plant-Based Sources:** Vitamin B12, primarily in animal products, requires supplementation for those adhering to a plant-based diet.

Consulting with Healthcare Professionals Before Taking Supplements

1. Tailored Health Assessments:

- **Existing Health Conditions:** Supplements may interact with conditions or medications; a healthcare professional's assessment identifies potential risks.

- **Nutrient Deficiencies:** Blood tests reveal deficiencies, guiding targeted supplement recommendations.

2. Potential Medication Interactions:

- **Prescription Medications:** Interactions with supplements may impact medication efficacy or cause adverse effects, necessitating professional guidance.

- **Balancing Act:** Healthcare providers ensure a delicate balance between prescribed medications and supplements for optimal health.

3. Considerations for Age and Gender:

- **Women Over 50:** Individualized recommendations for women over 50 address age-specific nutritional needs.

- **Postmenopausal Health:** Supplements like calcium and vitamin D become critical for bone health in postmenopausal women.

4. Pregnancy and Breastfeeding:

- **Folic Acid:** Pregnancy may require additional folic acid; healthcare professionals guide appropriate dosages.

- **Omega-3 Fatty Acids:** Essential for fetal development, supplements may be recommended during pregnancy and breastfeeding.

5. Regular Monitoring and Adjustments:

- **Periodic Check-ups:** Regular follow-ups allow monitoring of nutritional status, with adjustments to supplements based on changing health needs.

- **Identifying Red Flags:** Healthcare professionals identify potential issues, such as excess supplementation leading to toxicity, for timely interventions.

The Balance Between Whole Foods and Supplements

1. Nutrient Absorption from Whole Foods:

- **Bioavailability:** Whole foods offer more bioavailable nutrients, enhancing the body's absorption and utilization.

- **Synergistic Effects:** Whole foods provide a spectrum of compounds working synergistically for holistic health benefits.

2. Role of a Varied Diet:

- **Dietary Diversity:** A diverse diet minimizes reliance on supplements, ensuring a broad range of nutrients.

- **Whole Foods Synergy:** Whole foods offer a holistic package of nutrients, fibers, and phytochemicals supporting overall health.

3. Addressing Nutrient Gaps:

- **Identifying Deficiencies:** Supplements fill nutrient gaps identified through blood tests, providing targeted support.

- **Temporary Support:** Supplements act as temporary support, addressing deficiencies while dietary adjustments are made.

4. Potential Risks of Excessive Supplementation:

- **Vitamin Toxicity:** Excessive intake, like vitamin A or D, can lead to toxicity; healthcare providers guide appropriate dosages.

- **Mineral Imbalances:** Oversupplementation of minerals may disrupt delicate balances in the body.

5. Tailoring Supplements to Dietary Patterns:

- **Vegetarian and Vegan Diets:** Individuals with specific dietary patterns, like vegetarianism, may require targeted supplements to address nutrient gaps.

- **Individual Preferences:** Healthcare providers accommodate individual dietary preferences, ensuring nutritional adequacy.

Chapter 9

Bonus: 7-Day Cancer Diet Meal Plan

Welcome to an exclusive bonus chapter within the pages of "Cancer Diet Cookbook for Women Over 50." In this special segment, we present a meticulously designed 7-day meal plan crafted to align seamlessly with a cancer-conscious diet. Each day unfolds with a carefully curated selection of breakfasts, lunches, dinners, and snacks, ensuring not only nutritional richness but also delightful flavors. Furthermore, accompanying each meal is a detailed recipe, complete with essential nutritional information. To further support your culinary journey, we provide a comprehensive shopping list encompassing all the ingredients you'll need for the entire week. Join us on this week-long exploration of nourishing and delectable meals tailored to the needs of women over 50.

Day-wise Meal Plan with Breakfast, Lunch, Dinner, and Snacks

Day 1:

Breakfast: Nutrient-Packed Quinoa Bowl
- Quinoa cooked in almond milk, adorned with a medley of mixed berries and a dash of chia seeds.

Lunch: Grilled Chicken Salad Extravaganza
- A vibrant ensemble of mixed greens, grilled chicken breast, cherry tomatoes, cucumbers, and a drizzle of olive oil vinaigrette.

Dinner: Culinary Symphony - Baked Salmon and Roasted Vegetables
- Salmon fillet seasoned with aromatic herbs, harmonizing with a colorful array of roasted vegetables.

Snack: Greek Yogurt Serenade with Walnuts
- Greek yogurt and walnuts unite in a protein-rich and satisfying snack duet.

Day 2:

Breakfast: Avocado Toast Ballet with Poached Eggs

- Whole-grain toast pirouetting with mashed avocado and poached eggs, seasoned to perfection.

Lunch: Lentil and Vegetable Sonata

- A hearty lentil soup with a diverse medley of vegetables, creating a melodic midday meal.

Dinner: Turkey and Quinoa Crescendo - Stuffed Bell Peppers

- Bell peppers echoing with a melody of ground turkey, quinoa, tomatoes, and spices, baked to perfection.

Snack: Apple Slices Waltzing with Almond Butter

- Apple slices and almond butter dance together in a balanced and energizing snack.

Day 3:

Breakfast: Berry Smoothie Bowl Overture

- A symphony of blended berries, spinach, Greek yogurt, and honey, orchestrated into a bowl topped with granola.

Lunch: Chickpea Salad Waltz

- A whole-grain wrap pirouetted around a chickpea salad, mixed greens, and a light dressing.

Dinner: Grilled Shrimp and Quinoa Rhapsody
- Quinoa harmonizing with a colorful ensemble of stir-fried vegetables and succulent grilled shrimp.

Snack: Carrot Sticks Salsa with Hummus Beat
- Fresh carrot sticks salsa to the rhythm of hummus in a crunchy and satisfying snack.

Day 4:

Breakfast: Oatmeal Opera with Banana and Almonds
- Oatmeal, an operatic composition cooked in almond milk, starring sliced bananas and a sprinkle of almonds.

Lunch: Spinach and Feta Stuffed Chicken Crescendo
- Chicken breast, the lead performer, stuffed with spinach and feta, and baked to perfection.

Dinner: Vegetarian Brown Rice Symphony
- Brown rice orchestrating a symphony of sautéed vegetables, tofu, and a flavorful soy-ginger dressing.

Snack: Cottage Cheese with Berry Harmony

- Cottage cheese in harmony with a medley of fresh berries for a protein-rich snack.

Day 5:

Breakfast: Whole Grain Pancakes Waltz with Blueberries

- Whole grain pancakes waltzing with fresh blueberries and a dollop of Greek yogurt.

Lunch: Quinoa and Black Bean Concerto

- Quinoa and black bean salad performing a concerto with corn, tomatoes, avocado, and a lime-cilantro dressing.

Dinner: Baked Cod and Sweet Potato Mash Serenade

- Cod fillet serenaded with aromatic herbs and baked, accompanied by a side of mashed sweet potatoes.

Snack: Trail Mix Sonata with Nuts and Dried Fruit

- A trail mix sonata featuring a mix of nuts and dried fruits for a satisfying and energy-boosting snack.

Day 6:

Breakfast: Veggie Omelette Allegro with Whole Wheat Toast

- An allegro of flavors in a wholesome omelette, featuring an array of vegetables and served with whole wheat toast.

Lunch: Mediterranean Quinoa Bow - A Mediterranean Overture

- Quinoa bowl performing a Mediterranean overture with cherry tomatoes, cucumber, olives, feta cheese, and a drizzle of olive oil.

Dinner: Grilled Chicken Skewers and Rainbow Quinoa Rondo

- Grilled chicken skewers orchestrating a rondo with a side of rainbow quinoa and grilled vegetables.

Snack: Yogurt Parfait Harmony with Granola

- Layers of yogurt, granola, and fresh fruit harmonize into a delightful and nutritious snack.

Day 7:

Breakfast: Chia Seed Pudding Interlude with Mango

- A chia seed pudding interlude with almond milk, enriched with fresh mango chunks.

Lunch: Broccoli and Chicken Stir-Fry Finale

- Broccoli and chicken stir-fry concluding with a soy-ginger sauce, performed over a bed of brown rice.

Dinner: Eggplant and Chickpea Curry Crescendo

- Eggplant and chickpea curry crescendoing with aromatic spices, presented with a side of quinoa.

Snack: Nut Butter Energy Balls Coda

- Homemade energy balls, the final coda, made with nut butter, oats, and a touch of honey for a wholesome snack.

Detailed Recipes and Nutritional Information

Quinoa Breakfast Bowl:

- **Ingredients:** Quinoa, almond milk, mixed berries, chia seeds.
- **Nutritional Information (per serving): Calories:** 350, Protein: 10g, Fiber: 8g, Fat: 5g.

Instructions: Cook quinoa in almond milk, top with mixed berries, and sprinkle chia seeds for added texture and nutritional benefits.*

Grilled Chicken Salad:

- **Ingredients:** Mixed greens, grilled chicken breast, cherry tomatoes, cucumbers, olive oil vinaigrette.
- **Nutritional Information (per serving): Calories:** 400, Protein: 25g, Fiber: 6g, Fat: 18g.

Instructions: Combine mixed greens with grilled chicken, cherry tomatoes, cucumbers, and drizzle with a light olive oil vinaigrette.

Baked Salmon with Roasted Vegetables:

- **Ingredients:** Salmon fillet, mixed vegetables, herbs.

- **Nutritional Information (per serving): Calories:** 300, Protein: 22g, Fiber: 5g, Fat: 15g.

Instructions: Season salmon with herbs, and bake alongside a mix of colorful roasted vegetables for a flavorful and nutritious dinner.*

Shopping List for the Entire Week

Proteins:
- Chicken breast
- Salmon fillet
- Shrimp
- Cod fillet
- Eggs
- Tofu

- Ground turkey

Grains:
- Quinoa
- Brown rice
- Whole grain bread
- Oats

Vegetables:
- Mixed greens
- Spinach
- Bell peppers
- Cherry tomatoes
- Cucumbers
- Sweet potatoes
- Broccoli
- Eggplant
- Broccoli

Fruits:
- Berries (blueberries, strawberries, raspberries)
- Bananas
- Apple
- Mango

Dairy and Alternatives:
- Greek yogurt
- Feta cheese
- Cottage cheese
- Almond milk

Legumes:
- Black beans
- Lentils
- Chickpeas

Nuts and Seeds:
- Walnuts
- Almonds
- Chia seeds

Herbs and Spices:
- Olive oil
- Soy sauce
- Ginger
- Garlic
- Cilantro
- Lime

Others:
- Whole grain pancakes mix
- Nut butter
- Honey
- Hummus
- Trail mix (nuts and dried fruits)

Conclusion

As we approach the final pages of this comprehensive guide, "Cancer Diet Cookbook for Women Over 50," we extend our gratitude for joining us on this enlightening journey. This cookbook transcends a mere compilation of recipes; it stands as a testament to the intricate interplay between nutrition, lifestyle, and the pursuit of holistic well-being. Before we bid farewell, let's take a moment to revisit the key insights explored throughout this guide and then delve into offering encouragement for women over 50 to embrace a cancer-conscious lifestyle. Furthermore, we will equip you with valuable resources, ensuring that your journey toward health is supported by both knowledge and community.

Recap of Key Points

1. Understanding Cancer and Nutrition:

- Explored the profound connection between dietary choices and cancer risk.

- Discussed the vital role of inflammation, antioxidants, and phytochemicals in cancer prevention.

- Emphasized the need for a balanced and mindful approach to nutrition.

2. Tailoring the Diet to Women Over 50:

- Discussed the unique nutritional needs and metabolic changes in women over 50.

- Explored the impact of hormonal changes, particularly during menopause.

- Addressed common health concerns specific to this age group through dietary adjustments.

3. Explanation of How Diet Can Influence Cancer Risk and Progression:

- Delved into the intricate connections between dietary choices and cancer risk.

- Highlighted the significance of adopting a balanced and mindful approach to nutrition.

4. Key Nutrients and Antioxidants Essential for Cancer Prevention:
- Explored the role of specific nutrients like vitamin D, omega-3 fatty acids, and selenium.
- Discussed potential benefits of herbal supplements like turmeric and green tea extract.
- Emphasized the importance of probiotics for maintaining gut health.

5. Foods to Include and Avoid for a Cancer-Conscious Diet:
- Provided a detailed list of cancer-fighting foods, including fruits, vegetables, and lean proteins.
- Advised on the avoidance of processed foods, excessive red meat, and sugary beverages.
- Encouraged the consumption of a diverse range of colorful and nutrient-rich foods.

6. Bonus: 7-Day Cancer Diet Meal Plan:
- Offered a week-long meal plan complete with detailed recipes, nutritional information, and a shopping list.

- Ensured variety and flavor while adhering to the principles of a cancer-conscious diet.

- Facilitated a practical and enjoyable approach to incorporating healthy eating habits.

7. Understanding Supplements:

- Discussed the role of supplements in complementing a cancer-conscious diet.

- Emphasized the importance of consulting healthcare professionals for personalized recommendations.

- Explored the delicate balance between obtaining nutrients from whole foods and incorporating supplements.

Encouragement for Women Over 50 to Adopt a Cancer-Conscious Lifestyle

Embracing Change with Purpose:
Life beyond 50 is a dynamic and transformative phase, and adopting a cancer-conscious lifestyle becomes a powerful choice. Recognize the agency you possess in shaping your well-being and approach each step with intention. It's never too late to initiate positive changes, and every healthy choice is a testament to your resilience and commitment to a flourishing future.

Celebrate Progress, Not Perfection:
The journey towards a cancer-conscious lifestyle is a marathon, not a sprint. Revel in the small victories, whether it's choosing a vibrant salad over processed snacks or integrating a new nutrient-rich food into your diet. Progress is a sequence of small steps, and each one contributes to your overall well-being.

Nourishing Mind, Body, and Spirit:

A cancer-conscious lifestyle extends beyond dietary choices; it encompasses holistic well-being. Foster your mental and emotional health through mindfulness practices, engage in activities that bring joy, and prioritize restful sleep. Remember, true health emerges from the harmonious balance of mind, body, and spirit.

Community and Support:

You are not alone on this journey. Seek support from friends, family, or online communities that share your goals. Share your experiences, learn from others, and build a network of encouragement. A sense of community cultivates resilience and makes the journey more enriching.

Empowerment Through Knowledge:

Knowledge is a potent tool on your path to well-being. Stay informed about the latest research, nutritional insights, and lifestyle strategies. Empower yourself with knowledge, and let it be the compass guiding your choices toward a healthier, cancer-conscious lifestyle.

Resources for Further Information and Support

1. Cancer Organizations and Support Groups:

- **American Cancer Society (ACS):** Abundant information, support, and resources for cancer prevention and survivorship.

- **CancerCare:** Counseling, support groups, and educational resources for individuals and families affected by cancer.

- **Susan G. Komen:** A dedicated organization focusing on breast cancer awareness, education, and support.

2. Nutrition and Health Websites:

- **National Institute on Aging (NIA):** A valuable resource providing insights into healthy aging and nutrition for older adults.

- **Mayo Clinic - Nutrition and Healthy Eating:** A reliable source offering evidence-based information on nutrition, including tips for cancer prevention.

3. Cookbooks and Recipe Websites:

- **Cook for Your Life:** An enriching resource presenting cancer-conscious recipes and practical cooking tips.

- **Cancer Diet Cookbook for Beginners:** A comprehensive cookbook emphasizing the role of nutrition in both cancer prevention and recovery.

4. Fitness and Wellness Programs:

- **SilverSneakers:** A tailored fitness program designed for older adults, promoting physical activity and overall well-being.

- **AARP Fitness:** A platform offering a diverse range of resources, including workout videos and articles aimed at maintaining an active lifestyle.

5. Mindfulness and Mental Health:

- Headspace: A mindfulness app providing guided meditations for stress reduction and overall well-being.

- National Alliance on Mental Illness (NAMI): A resource offering support and information for mental health.

6. Government Health Websites:

- U.S. Department of Health & Human Services - Women's Health: An informative resource covering various aspects of women's health, including cancer prevention and nutrition.

Dear Reader, Did you enjoy this book? What are your thoughts? Kindly drop a review to share your impression of this book…….. Thanks

www.ingramcontent.com/pod-product-compliance
Lightning Source LLC
Chambersburg PA
CBHW050733260726
48661CB00001B/201